The Galveston Diet Revolution

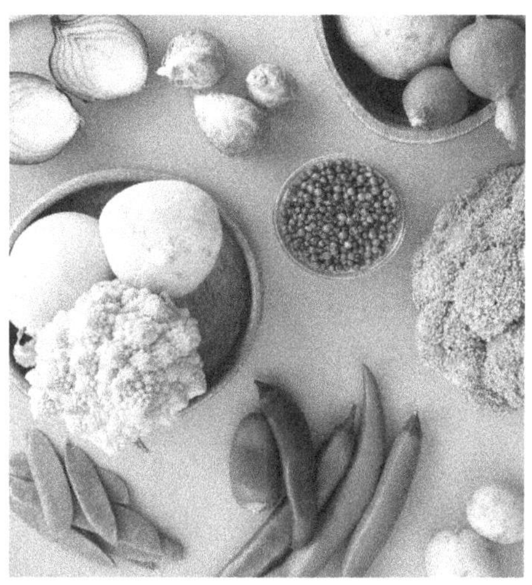

Unveiling the Secrets of Hormonal Balance for Lasting Results

Sylvia A. Stone

TABLE OF CONTENT

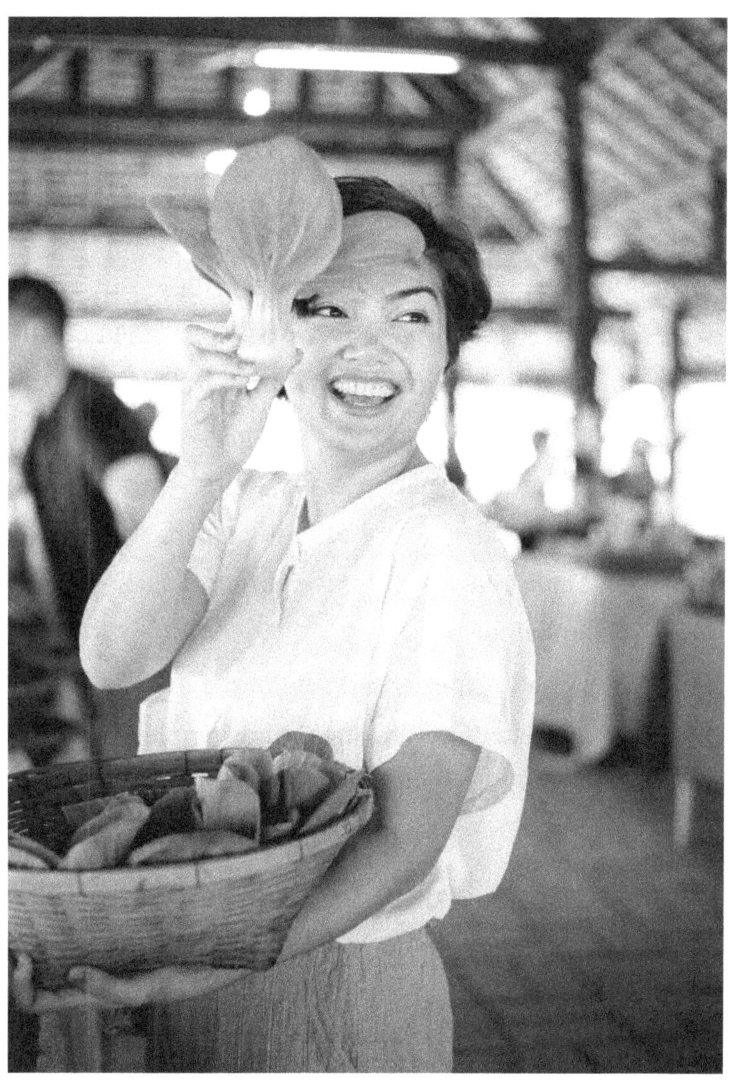

INTRODUCTION

1.1 The Origins and Principles of the Galveston Die

In a quaint coastal town, nestled by the shimmering waves of the Gulf of Mexico, lived a passionate and determined woman named Dr. Mary Claire Haver. As a respected physician, she dedicated her life to the care and well-being of her patients. But there was something more that fueled her desire to make a difference – her own personal journey with weight management and hormonal imbalances.

Dr. Haver had experienced the struggles of weight fluctuations, relentless cravings, and a rollercoaster of energy levels. She tried various diets and weight loss programs, only to find temporary results and a constant battle with her body. Frustration filled her heart as she witnessed the same challenges among her patients, especially women.

Determined to find a solution that would truly empower women and revolutionize their approach to health and weight loss, Dr. Haver delved deep into the realm of hormonal science and nutrition. It was during her exploration that she experienced a eureka moment – a realization that would change her life and the lives of countless others.

The Galveston Diet was born from Dr. Haver's passion, expertise, and the unwavering belief that women's health was intrinsically linked to their hormonal balance. Drawing inspiration from the beauty of her coastal surroundings and the nourishing bounty of the Mediterranean diet, she crafted a revolutionary approach to nutrition and wellness.

The Galveston Diet embraced the uniqueness of women's bodies and celebrated the transformative power of hormonal balance. It was a diet that went beyond mere calorie counting, promising a journey of self-discovery and a holistic lifestyle shift. Dr. Haver knew that the key to sustainable weight loss and improved well-being lay not in deprivation, but in nurturing the body with nutrient-dense foods and embracing a deeper understanding of hormonal harmony.

With every breakthrough in her research and each life she touched, Dr. Haver's passion only intensified. She became a beacon of hope for women seeking a new approach to health – one that celebrated their bodies and embraced the beauty of individualized nutrition.

Now, as you hold "The Galveston Diet Revolution" in your hands, you embark on a journey that transcends mere dieting. It is an odyssey of self-discovery, empowerment, and transformation. Within these pages lie the secrets to unlocking the potential of your body, revitalizing your energy, and achieving sustainable weight loss.

Welcome to a new era of health and well-being, where the power of science, passion, and a touch of coastal magic come together in the Galveston Diet. Prepare to embrace a revolution that will forever change the way you approach health and weight loss, as you become the author of your own transformative story. Let the journey begin.

1.1.1 *The Core Principles: Hormonal Balance and Sustainable Weight Loss:*

At the heart of the Galveston Diet lie two fundamental principles: hormonal balance and sustainable weight loss. Dr. Haver recognized that hormones played a pivotal role in metabolic regulation, fat storage, and overall health. By focusing on hormonal balance, she sought to create a transformative approach to weight loss that was sustainable, empowering, and embraced by women of all ages.

The Galveston Diet is not a quick fix or a restrictive regime; it is a comprehensive lifestyle change that celebrates the beauty of individualized nutrition and hormonal harmony. It encourages women to nourish their bodies with nutrient-dense foods, embrace intuitive eating, and cultivate a positive relationship with food – a powerful shift away from deprivation and towards self-care.

1.2 How the Galveston Diet Differs from Other Diets:

Unlike many conventional diets that overlook the role of hormones, the Galveston Diet stands apart with its unique and tailored approach.

1.2.1 A Focus on Women's Hormones and Individualized Nutrition:

The Galveston Diet recognizes that women's hormonal fluctuations, particularly during different life stages such as menopause, pregnancy, and perimenopause, can significantly impact weight management. Dr. Haver's personalized nutrition approach takes into account these variations, ensuring that women receive the specific nourishment needed to support their hormones and achieve optimal well-being.

By focusing on individualized nutrition, the Galveston Diet empowers women to understand their bodies better, identifying the specific foods that nourish and support their unique hormonal balance. This personalized approach provides a powerful foundation for sustainable weight loss and improved overall health.

1.2.2 The Importance of Long-Term Lifestyle Changes:

While many diets promise quick results, the Galveston Diet takes a different approach. Dr. Haver believes that sustainable weight loss and lasting health benefits can only be achieved through long-term lifestyle changes. Instead of a short-term fix, the Galveston Diet encourages women to adopt habits and practices that will support their well-being for years to come.

By embracing gradual changes and making thoughtful choices, women can establish a positive and lasting relationship with food and their bodies. The Galveston

Diet nurtures self-compassion, encouraging women to celebrate their progress and focus on the journey, not just the destination.

1.3 The Science Behind the Galveston Diet:

The Galveston Diet isn't just a concept born of passion and intuition; it is deeply rooted in scientific research and evidence.

1.3.1 Hormonal Imbalances and Their Impact on Weight Loss:

Scientific studies have established the link between hormonal imbalances and weight management. Fluctuations in hormones like estrogen, progesterone, and thyroid hormones can affect metabolism, appetite, and fat storage. The Galveston Diet addresses these imbalances through targeted nutrition, promoting hormonal harmony and facilitating sustainable weight loss.

1.3.2 Clinical Studies and Research Supporting the Galveston Diet:

The Galveston Diet has gained recognition and credibility in the medical community due to its evidence-based approach. Clinical studies and research have provided substantial evidence supporting the diet's effectiveness in improving hormonal balance, promoting weight loss, and enhancing overall health.

The Galveston Diet Revolution stands as a testament to the power of passion, dedication, and scientific foundation. Dr. Mary Claire Haver's journey and expertise have shaped a transformative approach to health and weight loss, one that goes beyond conventional diets and empowers women to embrace their uniqueness. By understanding the origins and principles of the Galveston Diet and the science that underpins it, women can embark on a life-changing journey of self-discovery, empowerment, and transformative health.

2.1 Getting Started with the Galveston Diet:

The Galveston Diet is a personalized and science-backed approach to weight loss and hormonal balance. Before diving into the phases and recipes, it's crucial to set clear goals and personalize your journey based on your unique needs and preferences.

2.1 Setting Goals and Personalizing Your Journey:

Start by defining your health and weight loss goals. Are you looking to lose weight, improve hormonal health, or enhance your overall well-being? Understanding your objectives will help you tailor the Galveston Diet to suit your specific needs.

Personalizing your journey involves considering factors such as age, activity level, and any pre-existing health conditions. Consulting with a healthcare provider or a registered dietitian can provide valuable insights and guidance on customizing the diet to support your individual requirements.

2.1.1 *Preparing Your Pantry: Essential Ingredients and Kitchen Tools:*

Creating a Galveston Diet-friendly pantry is essential for successful meal planning and preparation. Stock up on nutrient-dense ingredients that form the foundation of this diet. Some key items include:

- Chicken, turkey, salmon, tofu, and lentils are examples of lean proteins.
- Healthy Fats: Avocado, nuts, seeds, and extra virgin olive oil
- Brown rice, oats, quinoa, and whole-wheat products are examples of whole grains.
- Fresh Fruits and Vegetables: Berries, leafy greens, colorful veggies, and citrus fruits
- Herbs and Spices: Rosemary, thyme, turmeric, and cumin
- Kitchen tools like a blender, food processor, and quality cookware will make meal preparation easier and more enjoyable.

2.2 Phases of the Galveston Diet:

The Galveston Diet is divided into three distinct phases, each designed to optimize hormonal balance, support weight loss, and promote overall well-being.

2.2.1 Phase 1: Ignite:

Phase 1, also known as the Ignite phase, jump-starts your metabolism and sets the stage for successful weight loss. During this phase, you'll focus on specific foods and meal structures to regulate hormones and curb cravings.

2.2.1.1 Kickstarting Your Metabolism and Hormonal Balance:

The Ignite phase emphasizes consuming protein-rich meals to support lean muscle mass and stabilize blood sugar levels. Protein is essential for hormone synthesis and plays a crucial role in satiety, helping you feel fuller for longer periods.

Try a delicious breakfast recipe like the Galveston

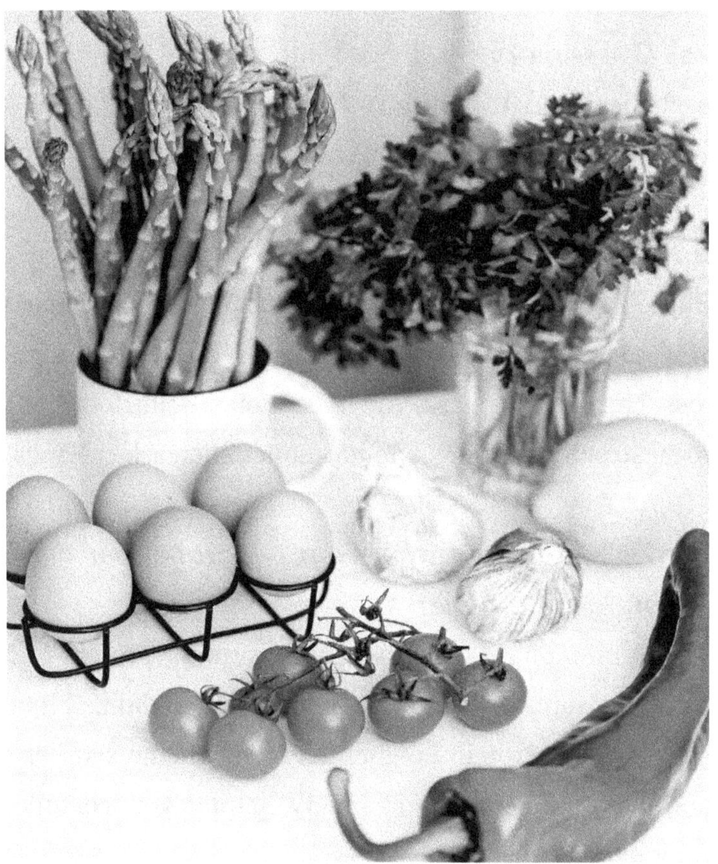

Ingredients:

- 3 large eggs
- 1 tablespoon of finely chopped fresh herbs, such as basil, chives, or parsley

- 1/2 cup diced vegetables (bell peppers, spinach, tomatoes)
- 1/4 cup shredded cheese of your choice
- Salt and pepper to taste
- 1 teaspoon olive oil

Preparation:

- Whisk the eggs with salt and pepper in a bowl.
- Heat the olive oil in a non-stick skillet over medium heat.
- Add the vegetables and sauté until tender.
- Once the eggs are set, pour them over the vegetables.
- Sprinkle the cheese and fresh herbs over the omelette.
- Fold the omelette in half and cook for another minute until the cheese melts.

Nutritional Value:

This omelette is rich in protein, providing essential amino acids to support hormonal health. The vegetables add fiber and a variety of vitamins and minerals.

2.2.1.2 Structuring Your Meals and Managing Cravings:

In the Ignite phase, you'll focus on three balanced meals and two small snacks per day to stabilize blood sugar levels and curb cravings. Structuring meals with adequate protein, healthy fats, and fiber-rich carbohydrates helps keep you satisfied and energized throughout the day.

A lunch recipe to try during this phase is the Galveston *Grilled Chicken Salad:*

Ingredients:

- 4 ounces grilled chicken breast
- Mixed greens (spinach, arugula, lettuce)
- Cherry tomatoes, halved
- Cucumber, sliced
- Avocado, diced
- 1 tablespoon balsamic vinaigrette dressing
- Optional: sprinkle of nuts or seeds

Preparation:

- Grill the chicken breast until fully cooked and seasoned to taste.
- Arrange the mixed greens, cherry tomatoes, cucumber, and avocado on a plate.

- Slice the grilled chicken and place it on top of the salad.
- Drizzle with balsamic vinaigrette dressing and top with nuts or seeds for added crunch and nutrients.

Nutritional Value:

This salad is a nutrient powerhouse, providing a balance of protein, healthy fats, and fiber from the greens and vegetables. The chicken offers lean protein, while the avocado contributes healthy monounsaturated fats.

2.2.2 Phase 2: Nourish:

After the Ignite phase, you'll transition to Phase 2, known as Nourish. This phase emphasizes a variety of nutrient-dense foods and encourages building balanced meals that sustain your energy and well-being.

2.2.2.1 Embracing Nutrient-Dense Foods and Building Balanced Meals:

During the Nourish phase, focus on incorporating a wide range of colorful fruits and vegetables, whole grains, and lean proteins into your daily meals. Essential vitamins, minerals, and antioxidants are present in these foods, supporting general health and vigor.

A nourishing dinner recipe is the Galveston Veggie *Stir-Fry:*

Ingredients:

- 1 cup mixed vegetables (broccoli, bell peppers, snap peas, carrots)
- 1/2 cup sliced mushrooms
- 4 ounces firm tofu, cubed
- 2 tablespoons low-sodium soy sauce or tamari
- 1 tablespoon sesame oil
- 1 teaspoon grated ginger
- 1 clove garlic, minced
- Optional: sesame seeds for garnish

Preparation:

- In a sizable skillet or wok set over medium heat, warm the sesame oil.
- Add the ginger and garlic, sautéing for a minute until fragrant.
- Add the mixed vegetables and mushrooms, stirring frequently until they begin to soften.
- Place the cubed tofu on the other side of the skillet after pushing the vegetables to one side.

- Drizzle the soy sauce over the tofu and cook until lightly browned on all sides.
- Combine the vegetables and tofu, tossing together until well mixed.
- Garnish with sesame seeds if desired.

Nutritional Value:

This veggie stir-fry provides a spectrum of vitamins, minerals, and phytonutrients from the colorful vegetables. The tofu adds plant-based protein, making it a satisfying and nutritious meal.

2.2.2.2 Exploring a Variety of Delicious and Satisfying Recipes:

The Nourish phase offers the opportunity to experiment with an array of delicious and nutritious recipes. Whether it's a nourishing smoothie for breakfast, a hearty grain bowl for lunch, or a flavorful curry for dinner, the Galveston Diet offers a plethora of options to keep your meals exciting and enjoyable.

Try the Galveston Green Goddess Smoothie for a refreshing and nutrient-packed breakfast:

Ingredients:

- 1 cup spinach

- 1/2 cup kale
- 1/2 avocado
- 1/2 cup frozen pineapple chunks
- 1/2 cup frozen mango chunks
- 1 tablespoon chia seeds
- 1 cup unsweetened almond milk
- Optional: honey or stevia for added sweetness

Preparation:

- In a blender, combine the spinach, kale, avocado, pineapple, mango, chia seeds, and almond milk.
- Blend until smooth and creamy.
- Taste and add honey or stevia if desired for added sweetness.

Nutritional Value:

This green smoothie is packed with vitamins, minerals, and antioxidants from the leafy greens and fruits. The avocado adds healthy fats, while the chia seeds provide omega-3 fatty acids and fiber.

2.2.3 Phase 3: Thrive:

Once you have successfully completed the Nourish phase, you'll enter Phase 3, the Thrive phase. Thrive is all about sustaining your progress, making lifelong lifestyle changes, and adopting a mindful approach to eating.

2.2.3.1 *Sustaining Your Progress and Making Lifelong Lifestyle Changes:*

In the Thrive phase, you'll continue to prioritize nutrient-dense foods while being mindful of portion sizes and hunger cues. Focus on incorporating a variety of foods into your meals, and continue exploring new recipes to keep your diet enjoyable and satisfying.

During this phase, you may notice that you have more flexibility in your food choices. You can occasionally enjoy your favorite indulgences in moderation without derailing your progress. However, remember that listening to your body and choosing foods that nourish and energize you will lead to the best outcomes in the long run.

2.2.3.2 *The Art of Mindful Eating and Enjoying Your Food:*

Mindful eating is a fundamental aspect of the Galveston Diet in the Thrive phase. It involves paying full attention to the eating experience, savoring each bite, and being present in the moment. Eating mindfully can help you recognize hunger and fullness cues, prevent overeating, and foster a healthy relationship with food.

For example, when enjoying a Galveston Dark Chocolate *Chia Pudding:*

Ingredients:

- 2 tablespoons chia seeds
- 1 cup unsweetened almond milk
- 1 tablespoon unsweetened cocoa powder
- 1 tablespoon honey or maple syrup
- 1/2 teaspoon vanilla extract
- Optional: fresh berries or sliced banana for topping
- **Preparation:**
- In a bowl, mix the chia seeds, almond milk, cocoa powder, honey or maple syrup, and vanilla extract.
- Stir well to combine all the ingredients.
- Cover the bowl and refrigerate for at least 2 hours or overnight until the chia pudding thickens.
- Serve chilled, topped with fresh berries or sliced banana if desired.

Nutritional Value:

This chia pudding is a delicious and satisfying treat with natural sweetness from honey or maple syrup. The chia seeds are rich in fiber and omega-3 fatty acids, promoting feelings of fullness and supporting heart health.

2.3 Customizing the Diet to Suit Your Needs:

One of the strengths of the Galveston Diet is its flexibility, allowing you to tailor the approach to your unique circumstances, preferences, and health conditions.

2.3.1 Adapting the Galveston Diet for Special Health Conditions:

If you have specific health conditions or dietary restrictions, the Galveston Diet can be modified to suit your needs. For example:

- **For individuals with diabetes:** Adjust carbohydrate intake and choose low-glycemic index foods to manage blood sugar levels effectively.

- **For those with food allergies or sensitivities:** Substitute allergenic foods with suitable alternatives while ensuring you still meet nutritional requirements.

- **For vegetarians or vegans**: Focus on plant-based protein sources like tofu, tempeh, beans, and legumes, and incorporate a variety of colorful fruits and vegetables for balanced nutrition.

- Consulting with a healthcare provider or registered dietitian can offer valuable guidance and support in customizing the diet to accommodate your health conditions.

2.3.2 *Tailoring the Diet to Your Food Preferences and Cultural Background:*

The Galveston Diet celebrates diversity and recognizes that cultural food traditions are an essential part of one's identity. You can tailor the diet to align with your food preferences and cultural background while still honoring the core principles of hormonal balance and nutrient-dense eating.

For example, if you enjoy Mediterranean cuisine, you can incorporate traditional dishes like grilled fish with olive oil, fresh vegetables, and aromatic herbs into your Galveston Diet meal plan. Similarly, if you love Asian flavors, you can experiment with stir-fries using a variety of colorful vegetables and tofu or lean proteins.

By adapting the diet to your culinary preferences, you'll find greater satisfaction in your meals and be more likely to maintain the Galveston Diet as a sustainable and enjoyable lifestyle.

In conclusion, the Galveston Diet is not just a temporary weight loss plan; it's a comprehensive lifestyle approach that empowers individuals to achieve hormonal balance, optimize their health, and make lasting changes in their lives. By understanding the different phases, incorporating nutrient-dense recipes, customizing the diet to suit individual needs, and embracing a mindful and balanced approach to eating, anyone can embark on a successful Galveston Diet journey and experience transformative results. The Galveston Diet is not just a diet; it's a transformational journey to a healthier, happier, and more vibrant you.

3.1 Key Nutritional Components of the Galveston Diet:

In the Galveston Diet, understanding and incorporating key nutritional components is vital for achieving hormonal balance and sustainable weight loss. This section delves deeper into the essential macronutrients, micronutrients, and phytonutrients that play pivotal roles in promoting overall health and well-being.

3.1.1 The Role of Macronutrients: Protein, Carbohydrates, and Fats:

Macronutrients are the fundamental nutrients that our bodies require in larger quantities to function optimally. The Galveston Diet emphasizes finding the right balance between these three essential macronutrients to support hormonal health and metabolic function.

3.1.1.1 Finding the Right Balance for Optimal Hormonal Health:

Balancing macronutrients is central to achieving hormonal balance. Dr. Mary Claire Haver emphasizes that an optimal balance of protein, carbohydrates, and fats is key to stabilizing blood sugar levels and regulating hormones, both of which are critical for weight management and overall well-being.

3.1.1.2 Protein as a Foundation for Lean Muscle and Satiety:

Protein plays a foundational role in the Galveston Diet, as it supports the development and maintenance of lean muscle mass, boosts metabolism, and enhances feelings of fullness and satiety. By incorporating adequate protein sources such as lean meats, fish, eggs, legumes, and dairy products, women on the Galveston Diet ensure their bodies have the necessary building blocks for healthy body composition.

3.1.1.3 Carbohydrates: Types, Timing, and Smart Choices:

Carbohydrates are not demonized on the Galveston Diet. Instead, the focus is on making smart carbohydrate choices. Dr. Haver recommends incorporating nutrient-dense, fiber-rich, and low-glycemic carbohydrates, such as whole grains, fruits, vegetables, and legumes. These choices provide sustained energy and prevent rapid spikes in blood sugar levels, contributing to hormonal balance and weight management.

3.1.1.4 The Power of Healthy Fats in Hormonal Regulation:

Healthy fats are another essential component of the Galveston Diet. Found in avocados, nuts, seeds, olive oil, and fatty fish, healthy fats play a crucial role in hormonal regulation, brain health, and nutrient absorption. Including these fats in the diet supports overall health and well-being.

3.1.2 Micronutrients: Vitamins and Minerals:

Beyond macronutrients, the Galveston Diet emphasizes the importance of consuming a wide variety of micronutrients, such as vitamins and minerals, to support overall health and hormonal balance.

3.1.2.1 Supporting Overall Health and Nutrient Absorption:

Vitamins and minerals are vital for supporting various bodily functions, such as immune support, energy production, and nutrient absorption. Consuming a diverse range of nutrient-rich foods ensures that women on the Galveston Diet receive a comprehensive spectrum of these essential nutrients.

3.1.2.2 Spotlight on Vitamins and Their Impact on Hormonal Balance:

Specific vitamins, such as vitamin D, B-vitamins, and vitamin C, play crucial roles in hormonal balance. For instance, vitamin D is essential for supporting thyroid function and immune health, while B-vitamins aid in energy metabolism and mood regulation. By understanding the role of these vitamins, women can make informed choices about their diet to support hormonal health.

3.1.2.3 The Vital Role of Minerals in Metabolism and Cellular Function:

Minerals, including calcium, magnesium, and zinc, are essential for healthy metabolism, bone health, and cellular function. By incorporating mineral-rich foods into their diet, women on the Galveston Diet support overall wellness and hormonal health.

3.1.3 Phytonutrients and Antioxidants:

Phytonutrients and antioxidants are powerful compounds found in plant-based foods, offering numerous health benefits and protecting the body from oxidative stress.

3.1.3.1 Harnessing the Healing Power of Plant-Based Compounds:

Phytonutrients are natural compounds found in fruits, vegetables, and herbs, known for their anti-inflammatory and immune-boosting properties. The Galveston Diet encourages the inclusion of a variety of colorful and diverse plant foods, allowing women to harness the healing power of these compounds.

3.1.3.2 The Immune-Boosting and Anti-Inflammatory Properties of Antioxidants:

Antioxidants, such as vitamins C and E, are powerful defenders against oxidative damage and inflammation. By consuming antioxidant-rich foods, women on the

Galveston Diet can protect their bodies from cellular damage and support overall well-being.

3.2 Creating Balanced and Nourishing Meals:

Applying the knowledge of the Galveston Diet's nutritional components, this section provides practical guidance on crafting balanced and nourishing meals that align with the diet's principles.

3.2.1 Breakfast Ideas:

Breakfast is considered a crucial meal on the Galveston Diet, setting the tone for the day and supporting hormonal balance. Dr. Haver offers energizing and hormone-supportive breakfast recipes that incorporate a balance of macronutrients, providing sustained energy and satiety.

3.2.1.1 Energizing and Hormone-Supportive Breakfast Recipes:

Some of the recipes include a hearty breakfast bowl with scrambled eggs, avocado slices, and sautéed spinach, providing protein, healthy fats, and essential vitamins and minerals. Another option is a nutrient-dense smoothie made with mixed berries, Greek yogurt, almond milk, and a tablespoon of flaxseeds, offering antioxidants, probiotics, and fiber.

3.2.1.2 The Art of Smoothie Building for Optimal Nutrition:

Smoothies are a versatile and convenient option for women on the Galveston Diet. Dr. Haver shares insights into the art of smoothie building, allowing women to customize their smoothies to their liking while ensuring they are nutritionally balanced. By combining leafy greens, fruits, protein sources like chia seeds or protein powder, and healthy fats like almond butter or flaxseed oil, women can create delicious and nutrient-packed smoothies.

3.2.2 Lunch and Dinner Recipes:

Lunch and dinner are opportunities to explore a diverse array of Galveston Diet-approved meals that nourish the body and delight the taste buds.

3.2.2.1 Flavorful and Filling Main Courses for Any Palate:

Dr. Haver presents a collection of delicious and filling main course recipes that cater to various palates while supporting hormonal health. Examples include a grilled chicken and vegetable skewer served with a Mediterranean-inspired quinoa salad, providing lean protein, fiber, and essential vitamins and minerals. Another option is a pan-seared salmon fillet with roasted vegetables, offering heart-healthy omega-3 fatty acids and an abundance of antioxidants.

3.2.2.2 Plant-Based and Protein-Packed Meals for Sustained Energy:

For women who prefer plant-based options or seek to reduce their meat consumption, the Galveston Diet offers a plethora of nutrient-dense plant-based meals. Dr. Haver includes recipes like a chickpea and vegetable curry with coconut milk, which provides a rich source of protein, healthy fats, and a variety of anti-inflammatory spices. Another plant-based option is a quinoa and black bean salad with avocado and lime dressing, offering a complete source of protein and an array of phytonutrients.

3.2.3 Snacks and Treats:

Snacks and treats are not excluded on the Galveston Diet. In fact, Dr. Haver encourages women to enjoy smart snacking choices that satisfy cravings and prevent overeating.

3.2.3.1 Smart Snacking Choices for Satisfying Cravings and Curbing Hunger:

Smart snacking is an essential aspect of maintaining energy levels and hormonal balance throughout the day. Dr. Haver presents a variety of satisfying and nutrient-dense snack options, such as a handful of mixed nuts, Greek yogurt with berries, or sliced vegetables with hummus.

3.2.3.2 Guilt-Free Treats That Won't Derail Your Progress:

Indulging in occasional treats is an important aspect of sustainable eating. Dr. Haver shares guilt-free treat recipes, such as dark chocolate-dipped strawberries or a banana-oat cookie made with natural sweeteners and whole ingredients. These treats offer a balance of flavors while keeping added sugars and unhealthy fats in check.

3.2.4 Sample Meal Plans for Each Phase:

To help women get started with the Galveston Diet, Dr. Haver provides sample meal plans for each phase of the diet: Ignite, Nourish, and Thrive.

3.2.4.1 Weekly Meal Plans for Ignite, Nourish, and Thrive:

The sample meal plans offer a clear and comprehensive breakdown of daily meals, including breakfast, lunch, dinner, and snacks, tailored to each phase's specific objectives. These meal plans ensure women receive balanced nutrition and support their hormonal health throughout their Galveston Diet journey.

3.2.4.2 Meal Planning Tips and Batch Cooking Strategies:

Meal planning is a key tool for success on the Galveston Diet. Dr. Haver shares practical tips and strategies to help women plan their meals efficiently, saving time and reducing food waste. Batch cooking is also encouraged to prepare larger quantities of meals that can be portioned and stored for later use, making it easier to stick to the Galveston Diet plan even on busy days.

Overall, the Galveston Diet is a scientifically grounded and nutritionally balanced approach to achieving hormonal balance and sustainable weight loss. By understanding and incorporating the key nutritional components of the diet, women can unlock the potential for improved well-being, increased energy, and a healthier relationship with food. The Galveston Diet empowers women to take charge of their health, making mindful and informed food choices that nourish both their bodies and minds. With practical meal planning, delicious recipes, and personalized guidance, Dr. Mary Claire Haver's Galveston Diet revolutionizes women's approach to nutrition and sets them on a path to long-term health and happiness.

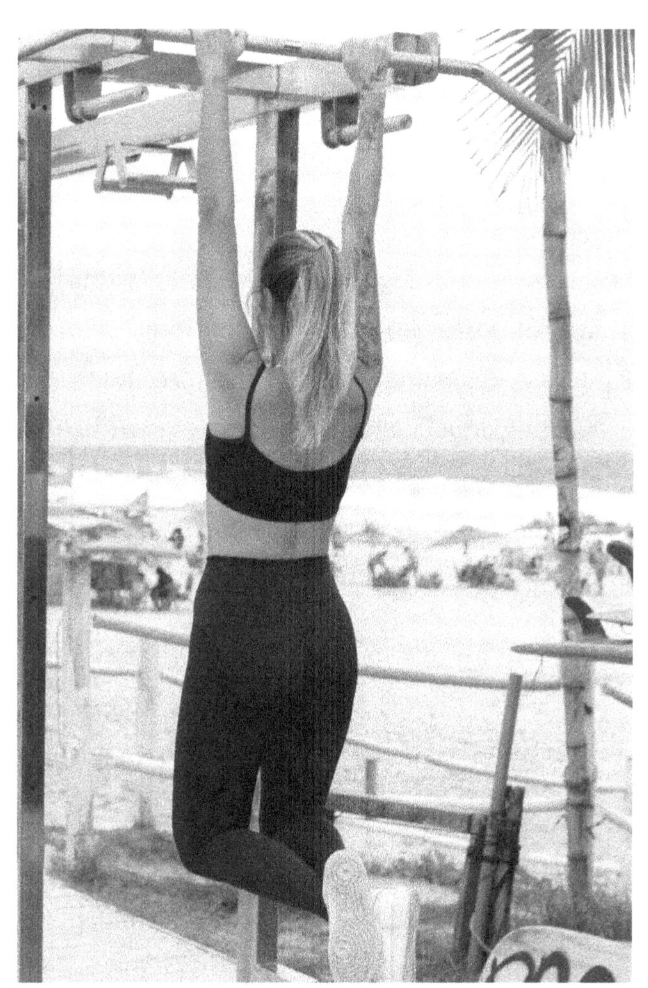

4.1 Incorporating Exercise and Physical Activity:

Regular exercise is an integral part of the Galveston Diet lifestyle, and it goes beyond just burning calories. Exercise plays a crucial role in maintaining hormonal balance, boosting mood, and improving overall health. Let's explore how exercise can be incorporated into your daily routine and how it positively impacts hormonal health.

4.1.1 The Synergy Between Exercise and Hormonal Balance:

Imagine starting your day with a brisk morning walk or a heart-pumping cardio session. As you engage in physical activity, your body releases endorphins, the feel-good hormones that elevate your mood and reduce stress levels. These endorphins act as natural stress relievers and contribute to a positive mindset throughout the day.

Now, let's consider the hormonal benefits of strength training. When you lift weights or engage in bodyweight exercises, your body responds by producing growth hormone, which is essential for tissue repair and muscle development. This hormone helps you build lean muscle mass, which not only improves metabolism but also enhances your body's ability to burn calories efficiently.

For example, a Galveston Diet follower named Sarah incorporates a mix of aerobic exercises and strength training into her routine. She enjoys morning jogs, cycling, and swimming for cardiovascular health, and she adds weightlifting and bodyweight exercises to her workouts to tone her muscles. Not only does Sarah feel physically stronger, but she also experiences increased energy levels and improved mood, all thanks to the hormonal benefits of her exercise routine.

4.1.2 The Best Types of Exercise for Weight Loss and Overall Well-Being:

The Galveston Diet encourages a diverse range of exercises to cater to different fitness levels and preferences. While cardio exercises like running, dancing, or cycling are effective for burning calories and improving cardiovascular health, strength training activities like weightlifting, bodyweight exercises, and resistance band workouts are vital for building lean muscle mass and improving metabolism.

Yoga and Pilates are excellent choices for individuals seeking low-impact exercises that focus on flexibility, core strength, and relaxation. These practices not only improve physical health but also have a positive impact on mental well-being. Sarah, from our earlier example, incorporates yoga sessions into her weekly routine to reduce stress and improve her flexibility, complementing her other workouts.

Moreover, the Galveston Diet lifestyle embraces outdoor activities like hiking, paddleboarding, or gardening, which provide both physical exercise and an opportunity to connect with nature. These activities not only contribute to physical fitness but also promote a sense of well-being and reduce stress levels.

4.2 Stress Management and Mental Well-Being:

Stress management is a critical aspect of the Galveston Diet lifestyle. Chronic stress can disrupt hormonal balance, lead to emotional eating, and hinder weight loss progress. Let's delve into how stress affects hormones and explore effective stress management techniques.

4.2.1 Understanding the Impact of Stress on Hormones and Weight:

The stress hormone, cortisol, is produced by your body when you are under stress. Cortisol is designed to help the body deal with stressful situations, preparing it for fight or flight responses. While this stress response is necessary in certain situations, chronic stress can lead to consistently elevated cortisol levels, affecting hormonal balance and metabolism.

For instance, when Sarah faces a particularly stressful workweek, she notices increased cravings for sugary and high-calorie foods. This is because cortisol stimulates appetite and encourages the body to seek out quick sources of energy. As a result, Sarah finds herself reaching for comfort foods to cope with her stress, leading to emotional eating patterns that hinder her weight loss progress.

4.2.2 Mindfulness and Meditation Techniques for Emotional Balance:

To effectively manage stress and promote mental well-being, the Galveston Diet encourages the practice of mindfulness and meditation. Being mindful means paying close attention to the present moment and objectively observing one's thoughts and feelings. By practicing mindfulness, individuals can develop a greater sense of awareness and learn to respond to stressors in a more balanced and composed manner.

Meditation, on the other hand, is a technique that focuses on quieting the mind, reducing mental chatter, and inducing a state of deep relaxation. Regular meditation practice has been shown to reduce cortisol levels and promote emotional balance, reducing the negative impact of stress on hormonal health.

For example, Sarah practices mindfulness during her meals. Before eating, she takes a moment to sit quietly, take deep breaths, and appreciate the food in front of her. By practicing mindful eating, Sarah can recognize her hunger and fullness cues more effectively, avoiding emotional eating and developing a healthier relationship with food.

Sarah also incorporates short meditation sessions into her daily routine, particularly during busy and stressful days. She finds that taking just a few minutes to meditate helps her to clear her mind, reduce stress, and regain focus, making her more productive and better equipped to handle daily challenges.

4.3 Sleep and Its Impact on Weight Loss:

Quality sleep is a critical component of the Galveston Diet lifestyle. Adequate sleep plays a vital role in hormone regulation, metabolism, and overall well-being. Let's explore the connection between sleep and hormonal health and discover tips for establishing healthy sleep patterns and routines.

4.3.1 The Connection Between Sleep Quality and Hormonal Regulation:

During sleep, the body undergoes essential processes of repair, restoration, and hormone regulation. Sleep helps to balance hormones responsible for appetite control, metabolism, and overall energy regulation.

For instance, when you experience a lack of sleep, your body's ghrelin and leptin levels may become imbalanced. Ghrelin is the hunger hormone that stimulates appetite, while leptin is the hormone that signals fullness. Sleep deprivation can lead to increased ghrelin production and reduced leptin production, resulting in heightened hunger and overeating.

Additionally, inadequate sleep can lead to insulin resistance, which affects the body's ability to effectively regulate blood sugar levels. This can contribute to weight gain and an increased risk of developing conditions like type 2 diabetes.

For Sarah, maintaining a consistent sleep schedule has been a game-changer for her weight loss journey. By ensuring she gets 7-8 hours of quality sleep each night, Sarah experiences improved energy levels, enhanced focus, and better appetite regulation, all of which support her efforts to maintain a healthy and balanced lifestyle.

4.3.2 *Tips for Establishing Healthy Sleep Patterns and Routines*:

To optimize sleep quality and support hormonal health, the Galveston Diet advocates for adopting healthy sleep patterns and routines. Here are some valuable tips for establishing a restful and rejuvenating sleep environment:

- *Create a Consistent Sleep Schedule*: Go to bed and wake up at the same time each day, even on weekends, to regulate your body's internal clock.

- *Create a Relaxing Bedtime Routine:* Develop a bedtime routine that promotes relaxation, such as reading, meditating, or taking a warm bath.

- *Avoid Stimulating Activities Before Bed:* Refrain from using electronic devices or engaging in stimulating activities close to bedtime, as these can interfere with falling asleep.

- *Create a Sleep-Conducive Environment*: Keep your bedroom cool, dark, and quiet to create an optimal sleep environment.

- *Limit Caffeine and Alcohol Intake:* Reduce or avoid caffeine and alcohol, especially in the hours leading up to bedtime, as these substances can disrupt sleep.

- By incorporating these sleep-enhancing practices into your daily life, you can improve sleep quality, optimize hormonal regulation, support weight loss efforts, and enhance overall well-being as part of the Galveston Diet lifestyle.

In conclusion, the Galveston Diet lifestyle encompasses more than just dietary choices. By incorporating exercise, stress management techniques, and prioritizing sleep, individuals can optimize hormonal balance, support weight loss, and improve overall well-being. By understanding the relationship between exercise and hormonal health, individuals can make informed choices about the types of activities that best suit their goals and preferences. Mindfulness and meditation practices provide valuable tools for managing stress and emotional eating, while improving sleep quality enhances hormone regulation and supports weight management. By adopting these lifestyle tips, individuals can embrace a holistic approach to health and well-being that aligns with the principles of the Galveston Diet, leading to lasting results and a more balanced and fulfilling life.

5.1 Navigating Social Events and Dining Out:

One of the common challenges individuals face when following the Galveston Diet is staying on track during social events and dining out. These situations often involve an array of tempting foods and can test your commitment to your health and weight loss goals. However, with the right mindset and strategies, you can enjoy these occasions while staying true to your plan.

5.1.1 How to Enjoy Social Gatherings While Staying Committed to Your Goals:

Social gatherings, such as birthday parties, family gatherings, and holiday celebrations, can be overwhelming with tempting treats and high-calorie dishes. However, with a few simple strategies, you can navigate these events without derailing your progress:

- **Eat Beforehand:** If you know that the food at the event may not align with your dietary preferences, have a healthy meal or snack beforehand to curb your appetite.
- **Focus on Socializing:** Instead of making food the center of attention, shift your focus to enjoying the company of friends and loved ones. Engage in conversations, play games, or participate in activities that don't revolve around food.
- **Bring a Dish:** Offer to bring a nutritious and delicious dish to the event. This way, you'll know there's at least one option that aligns with your dietary preferences.

For example, at a family gathering, John, a Galveston Diet follower, brought a colorful Mediterranean salad with fresh vegetables, olives, feta cheese, and a homemade vinaigrette. Not only did this dish impress his family, but it also provided him with a healthy and satisfying option to enjoy.

5.1.2 Making Wise Menu Choices at Restaurants and Special Occasions:

Dining out at restaurants or attending special occasions can present challenges in making healthy choices. However, with a little preparation and mindfulness, you can enjoy a delicious meal while staying true to your goals:

Check the Menu Ahead of Time: Many restaurants now offer their menus online. Take a look at the options beforehand, and choose a dish that aligns with the Galveston Diet principles.

Opt for Customization: Don't hesitate to request modifications to your meal, such as substituting fries for a side salad or asking for dressings and sauces on the side.

Portion Control: Restaurants often serve large portions, so consider sharing a dish with a friend or packing half of it to-go before you start eating.

For instance, when dining out with friends, Sarah follows these guidelines by ordering a grilled salmon salad with plenty of colorful vegetables and a light dressing. She enjoys her meal without feeling deprived and stays on track with her Galveston Diet journey.

5.2 Dealing with Plateaus and Setbacks:

Weight loss plateaus and setbacks are common on any health journey. While they can be frustrating, they are also opportunities for growth and progress.

5.2.1 Strategies for Breaking Through Weight Loss Plateaus:

Plateaus occur when your body adapts to your current diet and exercise routine, causing weight loss to stall. To break through a plateau, consider incorporating the following strategies:

Mix Up Your Workouts: Try new exercise routines or increase the intensity of your workouts to challenge your body in different ways.

Reevaluate Your Portions: Double-check your portion sizes and ensure you're not overeating, even on healthy foods.

Keep Hydrated: Sometimes, hunger and thirst can be confused. Drink plenty of water all day to avoid eating unneeded snacks.

For example, when Jane hit a plateau, she added high-intensity interval training (HIIT) to her exercise routine and focused on portion control. She soon began to notice progress once more.

5.2.2 Turning Setbacks into Opportunities for Growth and Progress:

Setbacks are a natural part of any journey, and it's essential to view them as learning experiences rather than failures. Use setbacks as opportunities to identify triggers, reassess your goals, and develop resilience:

Reflect on the Trigger: Identify what led to the setback, whether it was emotional eating, stress, or lack of preparation.

Adjust Your Approach: Learn from the setback and adjust your strategy accordingly. Maybe you need to plan better for social events or find alternative ways to manage stress.

Celebrate Your Progress: Remember to celebrate the progress you've made so far, regardless of setbacks. Each step forward is a testament to your dedication and effort.

For instance, when Sarah experienced a setback after a stressful week, she recognized that stress was a trigger for emotional eating. She decided to incorporate daily meditation sessions to manage stress more effectively and developed healthy coping mechanisms, ultimately helping her stay on track and overcome setbacks.

5.3   Finding   Support   and Accountability:

Having a support system and accountability can significantly impact your success on the Galveston Diet journey.

5.3.1 The Power of Community and Partnering with Like-Minded Individuals:

Joining a community of like-minded individuals can provide valuable support and motivation. Whether it's an online forum, social media group, or local meetup, connecting with others on a similar journey can make the experience more enjoyable and inspiring.

Sarah found a Facebook group of Galveston Diet followers where she could share her challenges and successes. The encouragement and advice from the group helped her stay motivated and committed to her goals.

5.3.2 Accountability Tools and Techniques for Long-Term Success:

Staying on track can be facilitated by accountability. Consider these techniques to hold yourself accountable:

- Journaling: Keep a food and mood journal to track your meals, emotions, and progress. This can help you identify patterns and make necessary adjustments.
- Buddy System: Partner with a friend or family member who has similar health goals. Check in regularly and offer each other support and encouragement.
- Set Specific Goals: Define clear and achievable goals, and regularly assess your progress. Celebrate your achievements and use any setbacks as opportunities for growth.

In conclusion, overcoming challenges and staying on track with the Galveston Diet requires dedication, adaptability, and a positive mindset. By navigating social events mindfully, managing stress, and prioritizing sleep, you can stay committed to your goals while enjoying a balanced and fulfilling lifestyle. Embrace plateaus and setbacks as opportunities for growth and continue making informed choices that align with the principles of the Galveston Diet. Surround yourself with a supportive community and use accountability tools to stay motivated and empowered on your journey to better health and well-being. Remember, it's the combination of mindful eating, regular physical activity, and a positive outlook that will lead you to long-term success on the Galveston Diet lifestyle.

6.1 Real-Life Testimonials of Galveston Diet Success:

The Galveston Diet has transformed the lives of countless individuals, leading to remarkable weight loss, improved health, and increased vitality. These inspiring success stories highlight the power of the Galveston Diet and the positive impact it has on people's lives.

6.1.1 Stories of Transformation and Empowerment from Galveston Dieters:

Susan, a 45-year-old mother of two, struggled with weight gain after having her second child. She tried various diets and exercise routines but found it challenging to sustain her progress. After discovering the Galveston Diet, Susan was drawn to its focus on hormonal balance and personalized nutrition. Within a few months of following the diet's principles, Susan shed excess weight, experienced increased energy levels, and improved her mood. She now feels empowered to make healthier choices and maintain her progress long-term.

John, a 58-year-old retiree, had struggled with chronic health issues for years, including high blood pressure and insulin resistance. When he started the Galveston Diet, he noticed a significant improvement in his health. His blood pressure normalized, and he was able to reduce his reliance on medication. The Galveston Diet's emphasis on nutrient-dense foods and balanced meals played a crucial role in John's health transformation, inspiring him to continue his journey to better well-being.

6.1.2 How the Galveston Diet Changed Lives and Improved Health:

Rachel, a 35-year-old professional, had been struggling with hormonal imbalances that affected her sleep and energy levels. After adopting the Galveston Diet, she noticed a remarkable difference in her hormonal health. Her sleep improved, and she experienced a newfound sense of energy and well-being. The Galveston Diet's science-backed approach to hormone regulation helped

Rachel regain control of her health and led her to advocate for the diet among her friends and family.

John, a 42-year-old father of three, had been overweight for years and felt self-conscious about his appearance. When he decided to try the Galveston Diet, he was amazed at how quickly he started losing weight. The diet's focus on whole, nutritious foods and portion control allowed him to shed pounds without feeling deprived. John's successful weight loss journey not only boosted his confidence but also inspired his family to adopt healthier eating habits.

6.2 Transformative Before-and-After Stories:

Pictures speak louder than words, and the before-and-after photos of Galveston Diet followers are a testament to the diet's effectiveness.

6.2.1 Witnessing the Amazing Results of the Galveston Diet in Action:

Before-and-after pictures showcase dramatic transformations, where individuals have not only lost weight but also improved their overall health. These stories often include visible changes in body composition, reduced waistlines, and radiant skin. The Galveston Diet's focus on sustainable weight loss through hormonal balance sets it apart from other diets, making it a popular choice among those seeking real and lasting results.

6.2.2 How Real People Achieved Their Goals and Thrived on the Galveston Diet:

Take Sarah, for example. She had struggled with yo-yo dieting for years and felt trapped in a cycle of losing weight only to gain it back. When she embraced the Galveston Diet, she discovered a new approach to eating that prioritized her health and well-being. Sarah lost weight steadily over several months and noticed significant improvements in her energy levels and mood. The Galveston Diet's emphasis on nourishing her body with whole foods and balancing her hormones allowed Sarah to break free from the cycle of dieting and develop a sustainable lifestyle.

These inspiring success stories are a reflection of the Galveston Diet's positive impact on people's lives. They show how a focus on hormonal balance, personalized nutrition, and long-term lifestyle changes can lead to transformative results. The Galveston Diet empowers individuals to take control of their health, embrace positive changes, and unlock their full potential for a happier and healthier life. Whether it's shedding excess weight, improving hormonal health, or gaining a newfound sense of confidence, these success stories serve as a powerful inspiration for anyone embarking on their Galveston Diet journey.

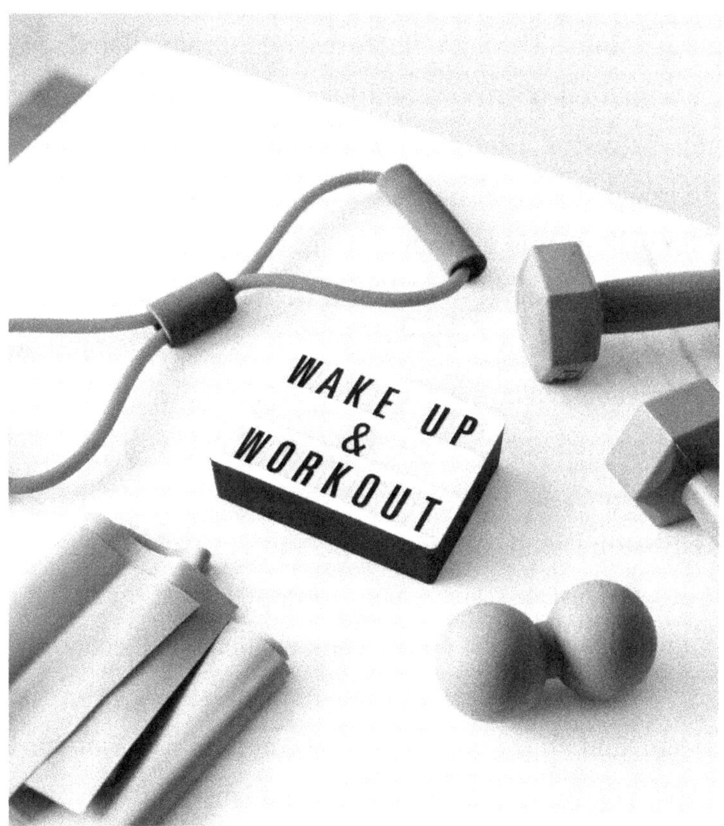

CONCLUSION

In conclusion, the Galveston Diet Revolution is not just a diet; it's a transformative lifestyle that empowers women to take control of their health and achieve sustainable weight loss. Through its focus on hormonal balance, personalized nutrition, and long-term lifestyle changes, the Galveston Diet has revolutionized the way women approach their well-being.

Throughout this journey, you have learned the origins and principles of the Galveston Diet, understanding how it differs from other diets and the science behind its effectiveness. You have discovered the power of setting personalized goals, preparing your pantry with essential ingredients, and embracing the three phases of the Galveston Diet: Ignite, Nourish, and Thrive.

The Galveston Diet has equipped you with the knowledge and tools to navigate challenges, incorporate exercise and physical activity, manage stress, prioritize sleep, and find support and accountability. You have explored the diverse range of delicious and nutritious recipes, understanding the importance of macronutrients, micronutrients, and phytonutrients in achieving optimal health.

As you embark on your Galveston Diet journey, remember that it is not just about the food on your plate but also about embracing a holistic approach to wellness. It's about nourishing your body with nutrient-dense foods, moving it with purpose, managing stress, and fostering a positive mindset.

By following the Galveston Diet, you are embarking on a life-changing experience that will not only help you achieve your weight loss goals but also enhance your overall health and well-being. It's a journey that will empower you to become the best version of yourself.

So, embrace the Galveston Diet Revolution with enthusiasm and commitment. Let it be the catalyst for positive change in your life. As you embark on this transformative journey, remember that your success lies in your dedication, perseverance, and belief in yourself.

Get ready to unlock your full potential, transform your body, and embrace a healthier, happier, and more vibrant life. The Galveston Diet Revolution awaits you. Take the leap, and let the magic unfold.

HEALTH IS WEALTH

ENJOY READING

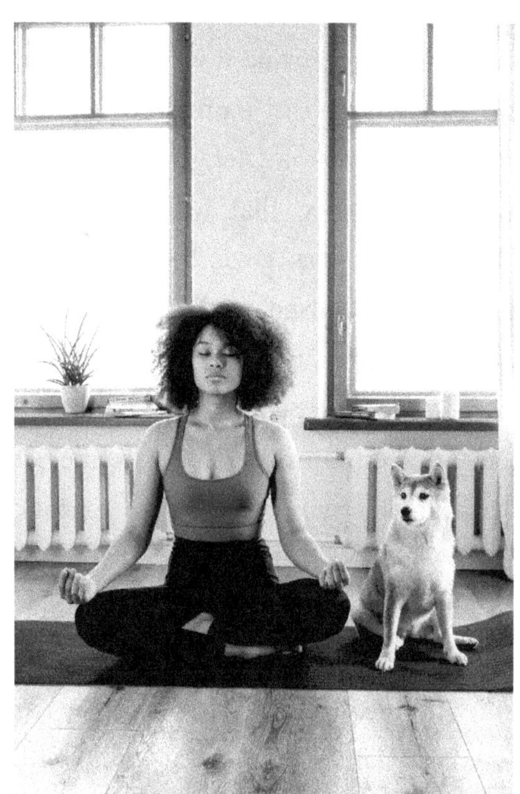